THIS FUCKING PLANNER BELONGS TO:

LET'S.

FUCKING.

DO THIS!

CANCER IS...
FUCKING BULLSHIT.

You're either going through this yourself or helping someone you love through this, so you know that already.

What you may not know, or may be becoming painfully aware of, is that cancer treatment is **also fucking bullshit**. You have to keep track of the endless medications, the rotating doctors and specialists in a variety of locations—all while you are experiencing fresh, new, fun-filled symptoms that you also need to monitor.

Keeping track of all this bullshit while *feeling* like bullshit is no easy task. Luckily, we are here to fucking help!

You need to focus on being a badass cancer warrior, not on the details of your day-to-day. Use this cancer tracker to defog your chemo brain and keep things running smoothly with your treatments as you rest and continue to kick ass.

Here's how to track your fucking symptoms and meds:

SYMPTOM, HABIT, OR MED	S	M	T	W	T	F	S
Drank Water!	X	X	X	X	X		
Headache				X		X	
Nauseous AF		X	X	X	X		
Hooray!! Food was eaten	X		X	X	X	X	

SUNDAY	MONDAY	TUESDAY	WEDNESDAY	THURSDAY	FRIDAY	SATURDAY

HEY, CANCER!

FUCK YOU,

YOU FUCKING FUCK!

THIS FUCKING WEEK

IMPORTANT CANCER SHIT

DAMN QUESTIONS TO ASK

TO DO

SHIT TO TRACK

SYMPTOM, HABIT, OR MED	S	M	T	W	T	F	S
_____							
_____							
_____							
_____							
_____							
_____							
_____							
_____							
_____							
_____							
_____							
_____							

WHAT FRESH HELL IS THIS?

MONDAY

TUESDAY

WEDNESDAY

THURSDAY

_____ / _____ / _____ TO _____ / _____ / _____

FRIDAY

SATURDAY

SUNDAY

THIS
WEEK'S
FUCKING
WINS

THIS FUCKING WEEK

IMPORTANT CANCER SHIT

DAMN QUESTIONS TO ASK

TO DO

SHIT TO TRACK

SYMPTOM, HABIT, OR MED	S	M	T	W	T	F	S
_____							
_____							
_____							
_____							
_____							
_____							
_____							
_____							
_____							
_____							
_____							
_____							

YOU'VE **FUCKING** GOT THIS!

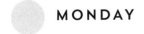 MONDAY

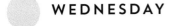 TUESDAY

WEDNESDAY

THURSDAY

_____ / _____ / _____ TO _____ / _____ / _____

FRIDAY

SATURDAY

SUNDAY

THIS
WEEK'S
FUCKING
WINS

THIS FUCKING WEEK

IMPORTANT CANCER SHIT

DAMN QUESTIONS TO ASK

TO DO

SHIT TO TRACK

SYMPTOM, HABIT, OR MED	S	M	T	W	T	F	S
_____							
_____							
_____							
_____							
_____							
_____							
_____							
_____							
_____							
_____							
_____							
_____							

KEEP CALM *AND*
KICK CANCER'S ASS

MONDAY

TUESDAY

WEDNESDAY

THURSDAY

_____/_____/_____ TO _____/_____/_____

FRIDAY

SATURDAY

SUNDAY

THIS WEEK'S FUCKING WINS

THIS FUCKING WEEK

IMPORTANT CANCER SHIT

DAMN QUESTIONS TO ASK

TO DO

SHIT TO TRACK

SYMPTOM, HABIT, OR MED	S	M	T	W	T	F	S
_____							
_____							
_____							
_____							
_____							
_____							
_____							
_____							
_____							
_____							
_____							
_____							

FUCK. THAT. NOISE.

MONDAY

TUESDAY

WEDNESDAY

THURSDAY

_____ / _____ / _____ TO _____ / _____ / _____

FRIDAY

SATURDAY

SUNDAY

THIS
WEEK'S
FUCKING
WINS

SUNDAY	MONDAY	TUESDAY	WEDNESDAY	THURSDAY	FRIDAY	SATURDAY

THE CHEMO

MADE ME DO

THIS SHIT

THIS FUCKING WEEK

IMPORTANT CANCER SHIT

DAMN QUESTIONS TO ASK

TO DO

SHIT TO TRACK

SYMPTOM, HABIT, OR MED	S	M	T	W	T	F	S
_____							
_____							
_____							
_____							
_____							
_____							
_____							
_____							
_____							
_____							
_____							
_____							

SEIZE THE DAMN DAY
(OR NOT & TAKE A FUCKING NAP)

MONDAY

TUESDAY

WEDNESDAY

THURSDAY

_____ / _____ / _____ TO _____ / _____ / _____

FRIDAY

SATURDAY

SUNDAY

THIS WEEK'S FUCKING WINS

THIS FUCKING WEEK

IMPORTANT CANCER SHIT

DAMN QUESTIONS TO ASK

TO DO

SHIT TO TRACK

SYMPTOM, HABIT, OR MED	S	M	T	W	T	F	S
_____							
_____							
_____							
_____							
_____							
_____							
_____							
_____							
_____							
_____							
_____							
_____							

OH, FOR FUCK'S SAKE!

MONDAY

TUESDAY

WEDNESDAY

THURSDAY

_____ / _____ / _____ TO _____ / _____ / _____

● **FRIDAY**

● **SATURDAY**

● **SUNDAY**

THIS WEEK'S FUCKING WINS

THIS FUCKING WEEK

IMPORTANT CANCER SHIT

DAMN QUESTIONS TO ASK

TO DO

SHIT TO TRACK

SYMPTOM, HABIT, OR MED	S	M	T	W	T	F	S
_____							
_____							
_____							
_____							
_____							
_____							
_____							
_____							
_____							
_____							
_____							
_____							

ONE DAY AT A FUCKING TIME

○ **MONDAY**

○ **TUESDAY**

○ **WEDNESDAY**

○ **THURSDAY**

____/____/____ TO ____/____/____

FRIDAY

SATURDAY

SUNDAY

THIS
WEEK'S
FUCKING
WINS

THIS FUCKING WEEK

IMPORTANT CANCER SHIT

DAMN QUESTIONS TO ASK

TO DO

SHIT TO TRACK

SYMPTOM, HABIT, OR MED	S	M	T	W	T	F	S
_____							
_____							
_____							
_____							
_____							
_____							
_____							
_____							
_____							
_____							
_____							
_____							

HOPE IS NOT FUCKING CANCELED

MONDAY

TUESDAY

WEDNESDAY

THURSDAY

_____/_____/_____ TO _____/_____/_____

FRIDAY

SATURDAY

SUNDAY

THIS WEEK'S FUCKING WINS

SUNDAY	MONDAY	TUESDAY	WEDNESDAY	THURSDAY	FRIDAY	SATURDAY

FIGHT LIKE A FUCKING BOSS

THIS FUCKING WEEK

IMPORTANT CANCER SHIT

DAMN QUESTIONS TO ASK

TO DO

SHIT TO TRACK

SYMPTOM, HABIT, OR MED   S   M   T   W   T   F   S

_____

_____

_____

_____

_____

_____

_____

_____

_____

_____

_____

_____

MONDAY

TUESDAY

WEDNESDAY

THURSDAY

_____/_____/_____ TO _____/_____/_____

FRIDAY

SATURDAY

SUNDAY

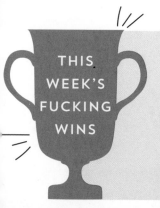

THIS WEEK'S FUCKING WINS

THIS FUCKING WEEK

IMPORTANT CANCER SHIT

DAMN QUESTIONS TO ASK

TO DO

SHIT TO TRACK

SYMPTOM, HABIT, OR MED	S	M	T	W	T	F	S
_____							
_____							
_____							
_____							
_____							
_____							
_____							
_____							
_____							
_____							
_____							
_____							

GIVE CANCER HELL!

○ **MONDAY**

○ **TUESDAY**

○ **WEDNESDAY**

○ **THURSDAY**

_____ / _____ / _____ TO _____ / _____ / _____

FRIDAY

SATURDAY

SUNDAY

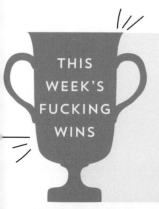

THIS
WEEK'S
FUCKING
WINS

THIS FUCKING WEEK

IMPORTANT CANCER SHIT

DAMN QUESTIONS TO ASK

TO DO

SHIT TO TRACK

SYMPTOM, HABIT, OR MED	S	M	T	W	T	F	S
_____							
_____							
_____							
_____							
_____							
_____							
_____							
_____							
_____							
_____							
_____							
_____							

IT'S OKAY TO
NOT BE FUCKING OKAY

MONDAY

TUESDAY

WEDNESDAY

THURSDAY

_____ / _____ / _____ TO _____ / _____ / _____

FRIDAY

SATURDAY

SUNDAY

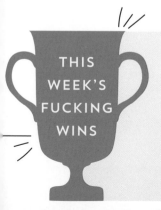

THIS
WEEK'S
FUCKING
WINS

THIS FUCKING WEEK

IMPORTANT CANCER SHIT

DAMN QUESTIONS TO ASK

TO DO

SHIT TO TRACK

SYMPTOM, HABIT, OR MED	S	M	T	W	T	F	S
_____							
_____							
_____							
_____							
_____							
_____							
_____							
_____							
_____							
_____							
_____							
_____							

A NEW, FUCKED UP SIDE EFFECT? WHY THE HELL NOT.

MONDAY

TUESDAY

WEDNESDAY

THURSDAY

_____ / _____ / _____ TO _____ / _____ / _____

FRIDAY

SATURDAY

SUNDAY

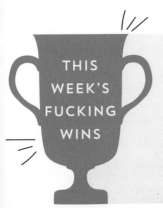

THIS
WEEK'S
FUCKING
WINS

THIS FUCKING WEEK

IMPORTANT CANCER SHIT

DAMN QUESTIONS TO ASK

TO DO

SHIT TO TRACK

SYMPTOM, HABIT, OR MED	S	M	T	W	T	F	S
_____							
_____							
_____							
_____							
_____							
_____							
_____							
_____							
_____							
_____							
_____							
_____							

IT'S FUCK-THIS-SHIT O'CLOCK

MONDAY

TUESDAY

WEDNESDAY

THURSDAY

_____ / _____ / _____ TO _____ / _____ / _____

FRIDAY

SATURDAY

SUNDAY

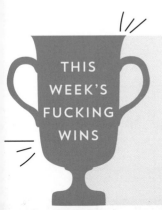

THIS
WEEK'S
FUCKING
WINS

MONTH & YEAR:

SUNDAY	MONDAY	TUESDAY	WEDNESDAY	THURSDAY	FRIDAY	SATURDAY

CANCER,
YOU PICKED
THE WRONG
BITCH

THIS FUCKING WEEK

IMPORTANT CANCER SHIT

DAMN QUESTIONS TO ASK

TO DO

SHIT TO TRACK

SYMPTOM, HABIT, OR MED	S	M	T	W	T	F	S
_____							
_____							
_____							
_____							
_____							
_____							
_____							
_____							
_____							
_____							
_____							
_____							

YOU *MAGNIFICENT* MOTHERFUCKER

MONDAY

TUESDAY

WEDNESDAY

THURSDAY

_____ / _____ / _____ TO _____ / _____ / _____

FRIDAY

SATURDAY

SUNDAY

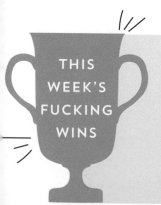

THIS
WEEK'S
FUCKING
WINS

THIS FUCKING WEEK

IMPORTANT CANCER SHIT

DAMN QUESTIONS TO ASK

TO DO

SHIT TO TRACK

SYMPTOM, HABIT, OR MED	S	M	T	W	T	F	S
_____							
_____							
_____							
_____							
_____							
_____							
_____							
_____							
_____							
_____							
_____							
_____							

PROBABLY TIME FOR
ANOTHER **FUCKING** PILL!

MONDAY

TUESDAY

WEDNESDAY

THURSDAY

_____/_____/_____ TO _____/_____/_____

FRIDAY

SATURDAY

SUNDAY

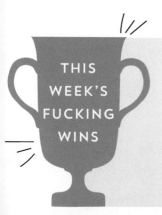

THIS
WEEK'S
FUCKING
WINS

THIS FUCKING WEEK

IMPORTANT CANCER SHIT

DAMN QUESTIONS TO ASK

TO DO

SHIT TO TRACK

SYMPTOM, HABIT, OR MED	S	M	T	W	T	F	S
_____							
_____							
_____							
_____							
_____							
_____							
_____							
_____							
_____							
_____							
_____							
_____							

IDK. IDC. IDGAF.

MONDAY

TUESDAY

WEDNESDAY

THURSDAY

_____ / _____ / _____ TO _____ / _____ / _____

FRIDAY

SATURDAY

SUNDAY

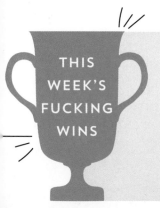

THIS
WEEK'S
FUCKING
WINS

THIS FUCKING WEEK

IMPORTANT CANCER SHIT

DAMN QUESTIONS TO ASK

TO DO

SHIT TO TRACK

SYMPTOM, HABIT, OR MED	S	M	T	W	T	F	S
_____							
_____							
_____							
_____							
_____							
_____							
_____							
_____							
_____							
_____							
_____							
_____							

WELCOME TO THE SHITSHOW

MONDAY

TUESDAY

WEDNESDAY

THURSDAY

_____ / _____ / _____ TO _____ / _____ / _____

FRIDAY

SATURDAY

SUNDAY

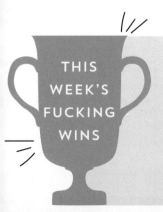

THIS
WEEK'S
FUCKING
WINS

SUNDAY	MONDAY	TUESDAY	WEDNESDAY	THURSDAY	FRIDAY	SATURDAY

SURRENDER?

NO

FUCKING

WAY!

THIS FUCKING WEEK

IMPORTANT CANCER SHIT

DAMN QUESTIONS TO ASK

TO DO

SHIT TO TRACK

SYMPTOM, HABIT, OR MED	S	M	T	W	T	F	S
_____							
_____							
_____							
_____							
_____							
_____							
_____							
_____							
_____							
_____							
_____							
_____							

YOU CAN *AND*
YOU FUCKING WILL

MONDAY

TUESDAY

WEDNESDAY

THURSDAY

_____ / _____ / _____ TO _____ / _____ / _____

○ **FRIDAY**

○ **SATURDAY**

○ **SUNDAY**

THIS WEEK'S FUCKING WINS

THIS FUCKING WEEK

IMPORTANT CANCER SHIT

DAMN QUESTIONS TO ASK

TO DO

SHIT TO TRACK

SYMPTOM, HABIT, OR MED	S	M	T	W	T	F	S
_____							
_____							
_____							
_____							
_____							
_____							
_____							
_____							
_____							
_____							
_____							
_____							

AND THERE GOES
THE LAST FUCK I GAVE

MONDAY

TUESDAY

WEDNESDAY

THURSDAY

_____ / _____ / _____ TO _____ / _____ / _____

FRIDAY

SATURDAY

SUNDAY

THIS WEEK'S FUCKING WINS

THIS FUCKING WEEK

IMPORTANT CANCER SHIT

DAMN QUESTIONS TO ASK

TO DO

SHIT TO TRACK

SYMPTOM, HABIT, OR MED	S	M	T	W	T	F	S
_____							
_____							
_____							
_____							
_____							
_____							
_____							
_____							
_____							
_____							
_____							
_____							

CRUSH THAT SHIT!

MONDAY

TUESDAY

WEDNESDAY

THURSDAY

_____ / _____ / _____ TO _____ / _____ / _____

FRIDAY

SATURDAY

SUNDAY

THIS WEEK'S FUCKING WINS

THIS FUCKING WEEK

IMPORTANT CANCER SHIT

DAMN QUESTIONS TO ASK

TO DO

SHIT TO TRACK

SYMPTOM, HABIT, OR MED	S	M	T	W	T	F	S
_____							
_____							
_____							
_____							
_____							
_____							
_____							
_____							
_____							
_____							
_____							
_____							

ORGANIZED FUCKING CHAOS

MONDAY

TUESDAY

WEDNESDAY

THURSDAY

_____ / _____ / _____ TO _____ / _____ / _____

FRIDAY

SATURDAY

SUNDAY

THIS WEEK'S FUCKING WINS

THIS FUCKING WEEK

IMPORTANT CANCER SHIT

DAMN QUESTIONS TO ASK

TO DO

SHIT TO TRACK

SYMPTOM, HABIT, OR MED	S	M	T	W	T	F	S
_____							
_____							
_____							
_____							
_____							
_____							
_____							
_____							
_____							
_____							
_____							
_____							

DON'T FUCKING PANIC

MONDAY

TUESDAY

WEDNESDAY

THURSDAY

_____ / _____ / _____ TO _____ / _____ / _____

FRIDAY

SATURDAY

SUNDAY

THIS WEEK'S FUCKING WINS

MONTH & YEAR:

SUNDAY	MONDAY	TUESDAY	WEDNESDAY	THURSDAY	FRIDAY	SATURDAY

YOU ARE
STRONGER
THAN THIS
SHIT

THIS FUCKING WEEK

IMPORTANT CANCER SHIT

DAMN QUESTIONS TO ASK

TO DO

SHIT TO TRACK

SYMPTOM, HABIT, OR MED	S	M	T	W	T	F	S
_____							
_____							
_____							
_____							
_____							
_____							
_____							
_____							
_____							
_____							
_____							
_____							

C'EST LA FUCKING VIE

MONDAY

TUESDAY

WEDNESDAY

THURSDAY

_____ / _____ / _____ TO _____ / _____ / _____

○ **FRIDAY**

○ **SATURDAY**

○ **SUNDAY**

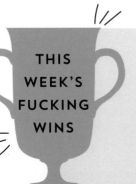

THIS WEEK'S FUCKING WINS

THIS FUCKING WEEK

IMPORTANT CANCER SHIT

DAMN QUESTIONS TO ASK

TO DO

SHIT TO TRACK

SYMPTOM, HABIT, OR MED	S	M	T	W	T	F	S
_____							
_____							
_____							
_____							
_____							
_____							
_____							
_____							
_____							
_____							
_____							
_____							

IT'S **OKAY** TO REST AND SHIT

MONDAY

TUESDAY

WEDNESDAY

THURSDAY

_____ / _____ / _____ TO _____ / _____ / _____

FRIDAY

SATURDAY

SUNDAY

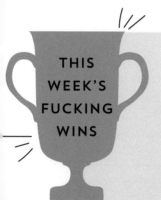

THIS
WEEK'S
FUCKING
WINS

THIS FUCKING WEEK

IMPORTANT CANCER SHIT

DAMN QUESTIONS TO ASK

TO DO

SHIT TO TRACK

SYMPTOM, HABIT, OR MED

S	M	T	W	T	F	S

WHAT. THE. **FUCK.**

MONDAY

TUESDAY

WEDNESDAY

THURSDAY

____ / ____ / ____ TO ____ / ____ / ____

FRIDAY

SATURDAY

SUNDAY

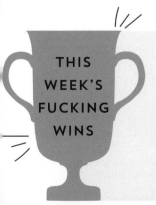

THIS
WEEK'S
FUCKING
WINS

THIS FUCKING WEEK

IMPORTANT CANCER SHIT

DAMN QUESTIONS TO ASK

TO DO

SHIT TO TRACK

SYMPTOM, HABIT, OR MED	S	M	T	W	T	F	S
_____							
_____							
_____							
_____							
_____							
_____							
_____							
_____							
_____							
_____							
_____							
_____							

BREATHE OUT THE BULLSHIT

MONDAY

TUESDAY

WEDNESDAY

THURSDAY

_____ / _____ / _____ TO _____ / _____ / _____

FRIDAY

SATURDAY

SUNDAY

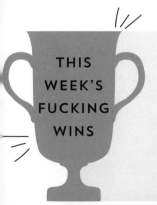

THIS
WEEK'S
FUCKING
WINS

SUNDAY	MONDAY	TUESDAY	WEDNESDAY	THURSDAY	FRIDAY	SATURDAY

BALD

&

BADASS

THIS FUCKING WEEK

IMPORTANT CANCER SHIT

DAMN QUESTIONS TO ASK

TO DO

SHIT TO TRACK

SYMPTOM, HABIT, OR MED	S	M	T	W	T	F	S
_____							
_____							
_____							
_____							
_____							
_____							
_____							
_____							
_____							
_____							
_____							
_____							

MONDAY

TUESDAY

WEDNESDAY

THURSDAY

_____ / _____ / _____ TO _____ / _____ / _____

FRIDAY

SATURDAY

SUNDAY

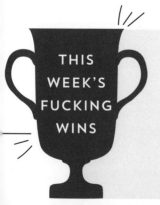

THIS
WEEK'S
FUCKING
WINS

THIS FUCKING WEEK

IMPORTANT CANCER SHIT

DAMN QUESTIONS TO ASK

TO DO

SHIT TO TRACK

SYMPTOM, HABIT, OR MED	S	M	T	W	T	F	S
_____							
_____							
_____							
_____							
_____							
_____							
_____							
_____							
_____							
_____							
_____							
_____							

BRAVE AS HELL

MONDAY

TUESDAY

WEDNESDAY

THURSDAY

_____ / _____ / _____ TO _____ / _____ / _____

FRIDAY

SATURDAY

SUNDAY

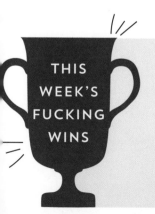

THIS WEEK'S FUCKING WINS

THIS FUCKING WEEK

IMPORTANT CANCER SHIT

DAMN QUESTIONS TO ASK

TO DO

SHIT TO TRACK

SYMPTOM, HABIT, OR MED

	S	M	T	W	T	F	S

_____

_____

_____

_____

_____

_____

_____

_____

_____

_____

_____

_____

SUPER FUCKING DUPER

MONDAY

TUESDAY

WEDNESDAY

THURSDAY

_____ / _____ / _____ TO _____ / _____ / _____

FRIDAY

SATURDAY

SUNDAY

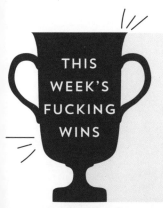

THIS WEEK'S FUCKING WINS

THIS FUCKING WEEK

IMPORTANT CANCER SHIT

DAMN QUESTIONS TO ASK

TO DO

SHIT TO TRACK

SYMPTOM, HABIT, OR MED

S	M	T	W	T	F	S

_____

S	M	T	W	T	F	S

_____

_____

_____

_____

_____

_____

_____

_____

_____

_____

_____

DON'T SWEAT THE SHIT THAT ISN'T HELPING YOU *GET BETTER*

MONDAY

TUESDAY

WEDNESDAY

THURSDAY

_____ / _____ / _____ TO _____ / _____ / _____

FRIDAY

SATURDAY

SUNDAY

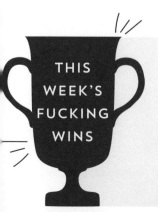

THIS
WEEK'S
FUCKING
WINS

THIS FUCKING WEEK

IMPORTANT CANCER SHIT

DAMN QUESTIONS TO ASK

TO DO

SHIT TO TRACK

SYMPTOM, HABIT, OR MED	S	M	T	W	T	F	S
_____							
_____							
_____							
_____							
_____							
_____							
_____							
_____							
_____							
_____							
_____							
_____							

YOU'RE. FUCKING. RADIANT.

MONDAY

TUESDAY

WEDNESDAY

THURSDAY

_____ / _____ / _____ TO _____ / _____ / _____

FRIDAY

SATURDAY

SUNDAY

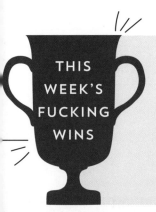

THIS WEEK'S FUCKING WINS

SUNDAY	MONDAY	TUESDAY	WEDNESDAY	THURSDAY	FRIDAY	SATURDAY

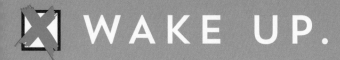 WAKE UP.

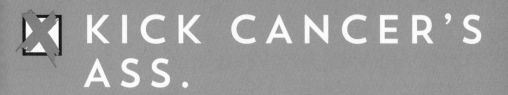 KICK CANCER'S ASS.

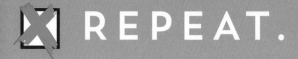 REPEAT.

THIS FUCKING WEEK

IMPORTANT CANCER SHIT

DAMN QUESTIONS TO ASK

TO DO

SHIT TO TRACK

SYMPTOM, HABIT, OR MED	S	M	T	W	T	F	S
_____							
_____							
_____							
_____							
_____							
_____							
_____							
_____							
_____							
_____							
_____							
_____							

BADASSES SHINE BRIGHT

MONDAY

TUESDAY

WEDNESDAY

THURSDAY

_____ / _____ / _____ TO _____ / _____ / _____

FRIDAY

SATURDAY

SUNDAY

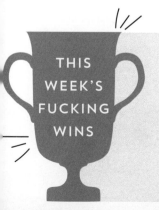

THIS
WEEK'S
FUCKING
WINS

THIS FUCKING WEEK

IMPORTANT CANCER SHIT

DAMN QUESTIONS TO ASK

TO DO

SHIT TO TRACK

SYMPTOM, HABIT, OR MED	S	M	T	W	T	F	S
_____							
_____							
_____							
_____							
_____							
_____							
_____							
_____							
_____							
_____							
_____							
_____							

FAN-FUCKING-*TASTIC*

MONDAY

TUESDAY

WEDNESDAY

THURSDAY

_____ / _____ / _____ TO _____ / _____ / _____

FRIDAY

SATURDAY

SUNDAY

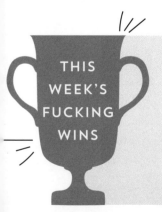

THIS WEEK'S FUCKING WINS

THIS FUCKING WEEK

IMPORTANT CANCER SHIT

DAMN QUESTIONS TO ASK

TO DO

SHIT TO TRACK

SYMPTOM, HABIT, OR MED	S	M	T	W	T	F	S
_____							
_____							
_____							
_____							
_____							
_____							
_____							
_____							
_____							
_____							
_____							
_____							

FUUUUUUUUUUUUUUUUUUUUUUUUUU UUUUUUUUUUUUUUUUUUUUUUUUUCK

MONDAY

TUESDAY

WEDNESDAY

THURSDAY

_____ / _____ / _____ TO _____ / _____ / _____

FRIDAY

SATURDAY

SUNDAY

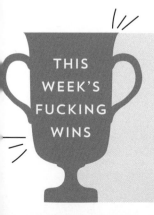

THIS
WEEK'S
FUCKING
WINS

THIS FUCKING WEEK

IMPORTANT CANCER SHIT

DAMN QUESTIONS TO ASK

TO DO

SHIT TO TRACK

SYMPTOM, HABIT, OR MED	S	M	T	W	T	F	S
_____							
_____							
_____							
_____							
_____							
_____							
_____							
_____							
_____							
_____							
_____							
_____							

EVERY DAY IS A
FRESH FUCKING START

MONDAY

TUESDAY

WEDNESDAY

THURSDAY

_____ / _____ / _____ TO _____ / _____ / _____

FRIDAY

SATURDAY

SUNDAY

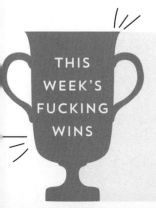

THIS
WEEK'S
FUCKING
WINS

SUNDAY	MONDAY	TUESDAY	WEDNESDAY	THURSDAY	FRIDAY	SATURDAY

A FUCKING WARRIOR, NOT WORRIER

THIS FUCKING WEEK

IMPORTANT CANCER SHIT

DAMN QUESTIONS TO ASK

TO DO

SHIT TO TRACK

SYMPTOM, HABIT, OR MED	S	M	T	W	T	F	S
_____							
_____							
_____							
_____							
_____							
_____							
_____							
_____							
_____							
_____							
_____							
_____							

WHEN IN DOUBT, SWEAR THAT SHIT OUT

MONDAY

TUESDAY

WEDNESDAY

THURSDAY

_____ / _____ / _____ TO _____ / _____ / _____

FRIDAY

SATURDAY

SUNDAY

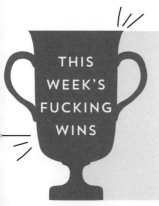

THIS
WEEK'S
FUCKING
WINS

THIS FUCKING WEEK

IMPORTANT CANCER SHIT

DAMN QUESTIONS TO ASK

TO DO

SHIT TO TRACK

SYMPTOM, HABIT, OR MED	S	M	T	W	T	F	S
_____							
_____							
_____							
_____							
_____							
_____							
_____							
_____							
_____							
_____							
_____							
_____							

FUCK *UNSOLICITED* MEDICAL ADVICE!

MONDAY

TUESDAY

WEDNESDAY

THURSDAY

_____ / _____ / _____ TO _____ / _____ / _____

FRIDAY

SATURDAY

SUNDAY

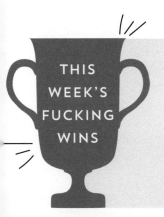

THIS
WEEK'S
FUCKING
WINS

THIS FUCKING WEEK

IMPORTANT CANCER SHIT

DAMN QUESTIONS TO ASK

TO DO

SHIT TO TRACK

SYMPTOM, HABIT, OR MED	S	M	T	W	T	F	S
_____							
_____							
_____							
_____							
_____							
_____							
_____							
_____							
_____							
_____							
_____							
_____							

ANYTHING IS FUCKING POSSIBLE

MONDAY

TUESDAY

WEDNESDAY

THURSDAY

_____ / _____ / _____ TO _____ / _____ / _____

FRIDAY

SATURDAY

SUNDAY

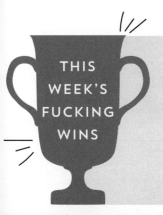

THIS
WEEK'S
FUCKING
WINS

THIS FUCKING WEEK

IMPORTANT CANCER SHIT

DAMN QUESTIONS TO ASK

TO DO

SHIT TO TRACK

SYMPTOM, HABIT, OR MED

	S	M	T	W	T	F	S
_____							
_____							
_____							
_____							
_____							
_____							
_____							
_____							
_____							
_____							
_____							
_____							

IT'S **OKAY** TO BE MAD AS HELL

● MONDAY

● TUESDAY

● WEDNESDAY

● THURSDAY

_____ / _____ / _____ TO _____ / _____ / _____

FRIDAY

SATURDAY

SUNDAY

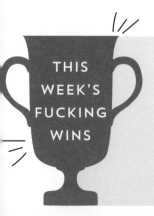

THIS
WEEK'S
FUCKING
WINS

MONTH & YEAR:

SUNDAY	MONDAY	TUESDAY	WEDNESDAY	THURSDAY	FRIDAY	SATURDAY

MAKE CANCER
YOUR
BITCH

THIS FUCKING WEEK

IMPORTANT CANCER SHIT

DAMN QUESTIONS TO ASK

TO DO

SHIT TO TRACK

SYMPTOM, HABIT, OR MED	S	M	T	W	T	F	S
_____							
_____							
_____							
_____							
_____							
_____							
_____							
_____							
_____							
_____							
_____							
_____							

YOU GLORIOUS BASTARD

MONDAY

TUESDAY

WEDNESDAY

THURSDAY

_____ / _____ / _____ TO _____ / _____ / _____

○ FRIDAY

○ SATURDAY

○ SUNDAY

THIS
WEEK'S
FUCKING
WINS

THIS FUCKING WEEK

IMPORTANT CANCER SHIT

DAMN QUESTIONS TO ASK

TO DO

SHIT TO TRACK

SYMPTOM, HABIT, OR MED	S	M	T	W	T	F	S
_____							
_____							
_____							
_____							
_____							
_____							
_____							
_____							
_____							
_____							
_____							
_____							

GO AT YOUR
OWN FUCKING PACE

MONDAY

TUESDAY

WEDNESDAY

THURSDAY

_____/_____/_____ TO _____/_____/_____

FRIDAY

SATURDAY

SUNDAY

THIS WEEK'S FUCKING WINS

THIS FUCKING WEEK

IMPORTANT CANCER SHIT

DAMN QUESTIONS TO ASK

TO DO

SHIT TO TRACK

SYMPTOM, HABIT, OR MED	S	M	T	W	T	F	S
_____							
_____							
_____							
_____							
_____							
_____							
_____							
_____							
_____							
_____							
_____							
_____							

HOT FUCKING MESS

○ MONDAY

○ TUESDAY

○ WEDNESDAY

○ THURSDAY

_____ / _____ / _____ TO _____ / _____ / _____

FRIDAY

SATURDAY

SUNDAY

THIS
WEEK'S
FUCKING
WINS

THIS FUCKING WEEK

IMPORTANT CANCER SHIT

DAMN QUESTIONS TO ASK

TO DO

SHIT TO TRACK

SYMPTOM, HABIT, OR MED	S	M	T	W	T	F	S
_____							
_____							
_____							
_____							
_____							
_____							
_____							
_____							
_____							
_____							
_____							
_____							

DON'T STOP FUCKING BELIEVING

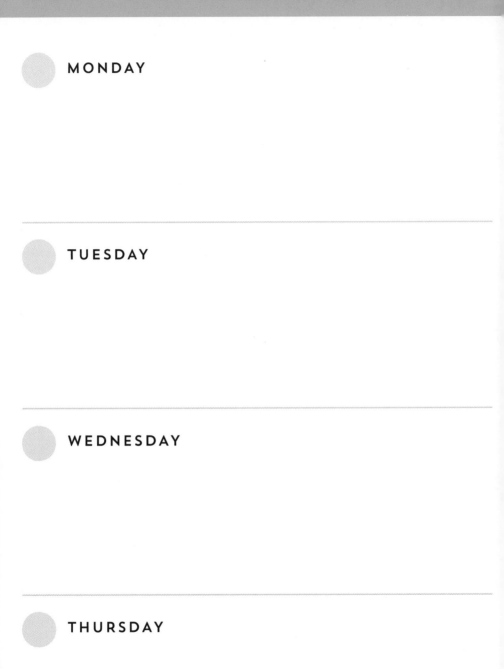

● MONDAY

● TUESDAY

● WEDNESDAY

● THURSDAY

_____/_____/_____ TO _____/_____/_____

● FRIDAY

● SATURDAY

● SUNDAY

THIS
WEEK'S
FUCKING
WINS

THIS FUCKING WEEK

IMPORTANT CANCER SHIT

DAMN QUESTIONS TO ASK

TO DO

SHIT TO TRACK

SYMPTOM, HABIT, OR MED	S	M	T	W	T	F	S
_____							
_____							
_____							
_____							
_____							
_____							
_____							
_____							
_____							
_____							
_____							
_____							

FRESH BULLSHIT SERVED DAILY

MONDAY

TUESDAY

WEDNESDAY

THURSDAY

_____ / _____ / _____ TO _____ / _____ / _____

FRIDAY

SATURDAY

SUNDAY

THIS
WEEK'S
FUCKING
WINS

SUNDAY	MONDAY	TUESDAY	WEDNESDAY	THURSDAY	FRIDAY	SATURDAY

CANCER FUCKING SUCKS

THIS FUCKING WEEK

IMPORTANT CANCER SHIT

DAMN QUESTIONS TO ASK

TO DO

SHIT TO TRACK

SYMPTOM, HABIT, OR MED	S	M	T	W	T	F	S
_____							
_____							
_____							
_____							
_____							
_____							
_____							
_____							
_____							
_____							
_____							
_____							

CAN'T TOUCH THIS SHIT

MONDAY

TUESDAY

WEDNESDAY

THURSDAY

_____ / _____ / _____ TO _____ / _____ / _____

FRIDAY

SATURDAY

SUNDAY

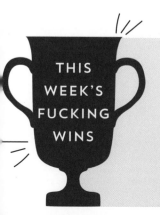

THIS WEEK'S FUCKING WINS

THIS FUCKING WEEK

IMPORTANT CANCER SHIT

DAMN QUESTIONS TO ASK

TO DO

SHIT TO TRACK

SYMPTOM, HABIT, OR MED	S	M	T	W	T	F	S
_____							
_____							
_____							
_____							
_____							
_____							
_____							
_____							
_____							
_____							
_____							

YOU'RE A FORCE TO BE
FUCKING RECKONED WITH

MONDAY

TUESDAY

WEDNESDAY

THURSDAY

_____ / _____ / _____ TO _____ / _____ / _____

○ **FRIDAY**

○ **SATURDAY**

○ **SUNDAY**

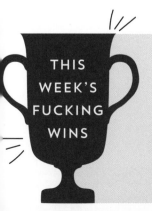

THIS
WEEK'S
FUCKING
WINS

THIS FUCKING WEEK

IMPORTANT CANCER SHIT

DAMN QUESTIONS TO ASK

TO DO

SHIT TO TRACK

SYMPTOM, HABIT, OR MED

	S	M	T	W	T	F	S
_____							
_____							
_____							
_____							
_____							
_____							
_____							
_____							
_____							
_____							
_____							
_____							

STRONGER
THAN FUCKING YESTERDAY

MONDAY

TUESDAY

WEDNESDAY

THURSDAY

_____ / _____ / _____ TO _____ / _____ / _____

○ **FRIDAY**

○ **SATURDAY**

○ **SUNDAY**

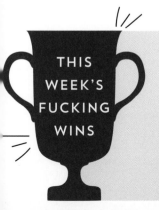

THIS
WEEK'S
FUCKING
WINS

THIS FUCKING WEEK

IMPORTANT CANCER SHIT

DAMN QUESTIONS TO ASK

TO DO

SHIT TO TRACK

SYMPTOM, HABIT, OR MED

	S	M	T	W	T	F	S
_____							
_____							
_____							
_____							
_____							
_____							
_____							
_____							
_____							
_____							
_____							
_____							

MONDAY

TUESDAY

WEDNESDAY

THURSDAY

_____ / _____ / _____ TO _____ / _____ / _____

FRIDAY

SATURDAY

SUNDAY

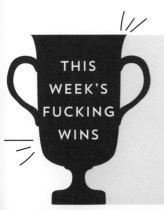

THIS WEEK'S FUCKING WINS

MONTH & YEAR:

SUNDAY	MONDAY	TUESDAY	WEDNESDAY	THURSDAY	FRIDAY	SATURDAY

TOUGH

AS

HELL

THIS FUCKING WEEK

IMPORTANT CANCER SHIT

DAMN QUESTIONS TO ASK

TO DO

SHIT TO TRACK

SYMPTOM, HABIT, OR MED	S	M	T	W	T	F	S
_____							
_____							
_____							
_____							
_____							
_____							
_____							
_____							
_____							
_____							
_____							
_____							

FOCUS ON BEATING THIS BITCH!

● MONDAY

● TUESDAY

● WEDNESDAY

● THURSDAY

_____/_____/_____ TO _____/_____/_____

● FRIDAY

● SATURDAY

● SUNDAY

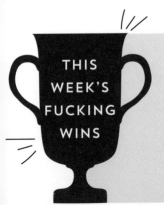

THIS
WEEK'S
FUCKING
WINS

THIS FUCKING WEEK

IMPORTANT CANCER SHIT

DAMN QUESTIONS TO ASK

TO DO

SHIT TO TRACK

SYMPTOM, HABIT, OR MED	S	M	T	W	T	F	S
_____							
_____							
_____							
_____							
_____							
_____							
_____							
_____							
_____							
_____							
_____							
_____							

WHAT YOU SEE IS
WHAT YOU FUCKING GET

MONDAY

TUESDAY

WEDNESDAY

THURSDAY

_____ / _____ / _____ TO _____ / _____ / _____

○ FRIDAY

○ SATURDAY

○ SUNDAY

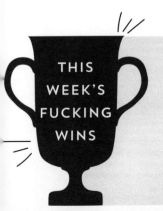

THIS WEEK'S FUCKING WINS

THIS FUCKING WEEK

IMPORTANT CANCER SHIT

DAMN QUESTIONS TO ASK

TO DO

SHIT TO TRACK

SYMPTOM, HABIT, OR MED	S	M	T	W	T	F	S
_____							
_____							
_____							
_____							
_____							
_____							
_____							
_____							
_____							
_____							
_____							
_____							

FUCK CANCER RIGHT IN
ITS STUPID FUCKING FACE!

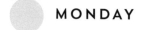 **MONDAY**

TUESDAY

WEDNESDAY

THURSDAY

_____/_____/_____ TO _____/_____/_____

FRIDAY

SATURDAY

SUNDAY

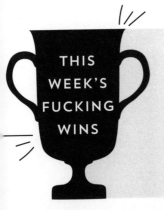

THIS
WEEK'S
FUCKING
WINS

THIS FUCKING WEEK

IMPORTANT CANCER SHIT

DAMN QUESTIONS TO ASK

TO DO

SHIT TO TRACK

SYMPTOM, HABIT, OR MED	S	M	T	W	T	F	S
_____							
_____							
_____							
_____							
_____							
_____							
_____							
_____							
_____							
_____							
_____							
_____							

FIGHT HARD, LIVE FUCKING WELL

MONDAY

TUESDAY

WEDNESDAY

THURSDAY

_____/_____/_____ TO _____/_____/_____

○ **FRIDAY**

○ **SATURDAY**

○ **SUNDAY**

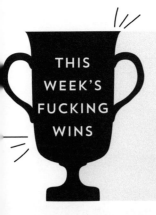

THIS WEEK'S FUCKING WINS

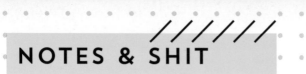

NOTES & SHIT

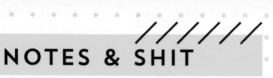

NOTES & SHIT

This planner was developed with cancer fighters, survivors, and badass caregivers who know just how much cancer fucking sucks.

YOU'VE FUCKING GOT THIS!

Published by Sourcebooks
P.O. Box 4410, Naperville, Illinois 60567-4410
(630) 961-3900
sourcebooks.com

Printed and bound in China.
OGP 10 9 8 7 6 5 4 3 2 1

SELF FUCKING CARE

KEEP FUCKING GOING

ANOTHER FUCKING DOCTOR APPT	ANOTHER FUCKING DOCTOR APPT	ANOTHER FUCKING DOCTOR APPT
ANOTHER FUCKING DOCTOR APPT	ANOTHER FUCKING DOCTOR APPT	ANOTHER FUCKING DOCTOR APPT
ANOTHER FUCKING DOCTOR APPT	ANOTHER FUCKING DOCTOR APPT	ANOTHER FUCKING DOCTOR APPT
ANOTHER FUCKING DOCTOR APPT	ANOTHER FUCKING DOCTOR APPT	ANOTHER FUCKING DOCTOR APPT
ANOTHER FUCKING DOCTOR APPT	ANOTHER FUCKING DOCTOR APPT	ANOTHER FUCKING DOCTOR APPT
ANOTHER FUCKING DOCTOR APPT	ANOTHER FUCKING DOCTOR APPT	ANOTHER FUCKING DOCTOR APPT
ANOTHER FUCKING DOCTOR APPT	ANOTHER FUCKING DOCTOR APPT	ANOTHER FUCKING DOCTOR APPT
ANOTHER FUCKING DOCTOR APPT	ANOTHER FUCKING DOCTOR APPT	ANOTHER FUCKING DOCTOR APPT
ANOTHER FUCKING DOCTOR APPT	ANOTHER FUCKING DOCTOR APPT	ANOTHER FUCKING DOCTOR APPT
ANOTHER FUCKING DOCTOR APPT	ANOTHER FUCKING DOCTOR APPT	ANOTHER FUCKING DOCTOR APPT
ANOTHER FUCKING DOCTOR APPT	ANOTHER FUCKING DOCTOR APPT	ANOTHER FUCKING DOCTOR APPT
ANOTHER FUCKING DOCTOR APPT	ANOTHER FUCKING DOCTOR APPT	ANOTHER FUCKING DOCTOR APPT
ANOTHER FUCKING DOCTOR APPT	ANOTHER FUCKING DOCTOR APPT	ANOTHER FUCKING DOCTOR APPT

ANOTHER FUCKING DOCTOR APPT

ANOTHER FUCKING DOCTOR APPT

ANOTHER FUCKING DOCTOR APPT

ANOTHER FUCKING DOCTOR APPT

ANOTHER FUCKING DOCTOR APPT

ANOTHER FUCKING DOCTOR APPT

ANOTHER FUCKING DOCTOR APPT

ANOTHER FUCKING DOCTOR APPT

ANOTHER FUCKING DOCTOR APPT

ANOTHER FUCKING DOCTOR APPT

ANOTHER FUCKING DOCTOR APPT

ANOTHER FUCKING DOCTOR APPT

ANOTHER FUCKING DOCTOR APPT

ANOTHER FUCKING DOCTOR APPT

ANOTHER FUCKING DOCTOR APPT

ANOTHER FUCKING DOCTOR APPT

ANOTHER FUCKING DOCTOR APPT

ANOTHER FUCKING DOCTOR APPT

ANOTHER FUCKING DOCTOR APPT

ANOTHER FUCKING DOCTOR APPT

ANOTHER FUCKING DOCTOR APPT

ANOTHER FUCKING DOCTOR APPT

ANOTHER FUCKING DOCTOR APPT

ANOTHER FUCKING DOCTOR APPT

ANOTHER FUCKING DOCTOR APPT

ANOTHER FUCKING DOCTOR APPT

ANOTHER FUCKING DOCTOR APPT

ANOTHER FUCKING DOCTOR APPT

ANOTHER FUCKING DOCTOR APPT

ANOTHER FUCKING DOCTOR APPT

ANOTHER FUCKING DOCTOR APPT

ANOTHER FUCKING DOCTOR APPT

ANOTHER FUCKING DOCTOR APPT

ANOTHER FUCKING DOCTOR APPT

ANOTHER FUCKING DOCTOR APPT

ANOTHER FUCKING DOCTOR APPT

ANOTHER FUCKING DOCTOR APPT

ANOTHER FUCKING DOCTOR APPT

ANOTHER FUCKING DOCTOR APPT

ANOTHER FUCKING DOCTOR APPT

ANOTHER FUCKING DOCTOR APPT

ANOTHER FUCKING DOCTOR APPT

FUCK CANCER

FUCK CANCER

FUCK CANCER

FUCK CANCER

FUCK CANCER

FUCK CANCER

FUCK CANCER

CAUTION: FUCKING RADIOACTIVE

CAUTION: FUCKING RADIOACTIVE

CAUTION: FUCKING RADIOACTIVE

CAUTION: FUCKING RADIOACTIVE

CAUTION: FUCKING RADIOACTIVE

CAUTION: FUCKING RADIOACTIVE

FUCK THIS

WTF

FUCK THAT

FML

FUCK THIS

WTF

FUCK THAT

FML

FUCK THIS

WTF

FUCK THAT

FML

F*CK CANCER

SHIT HAPPENS

SHIT HAPPENS

F*CK CANCER

F*CK CANCER

YOU GLORIOUS BASTARD (×9)

YOU'RE A GODDAMN ROCK STAR (×9)

BADASS BITCH (×9)

KICK SOME ASS (×9)

MAKE CANCER YOUR BITCH (×9)

CALM THE FUCK DOWN (×9)

ANOTHER FUCKING
DOCTOR APPT

ANOTHER FUCKING
DOCTOR APPT

ANOTHER FUCKING
DOCTOR APPT

ANOTHER FUCKING
DOCTOR APPT

ANOTHER FUCKING
DOCTOR APPT

ANOTHER FUCKING
DOCTOR APPT

ANOTHER FUCKING
DOCTOR APPT

ANOTHER FUCKING
DOCTOR APPT

ANOTHER FUCKING
DOCTOR APPT

GIVE 'EM
HELL

GIVE 'EM
HELL

GIVE 'EM
HELL

GIVE 'EM
HELL

GIVE 'EM
HELL

GIVE 'EM
HELL

GIVE 'EM
HELL

GIVE 'EM
HELL

GIVE 'EM
HELL

TIRED
AF

TIRED
AF

TIRED
AF

TIRED
AF

TIRED
AF

TIRED
AF

TIRED
AF

TIRED
AF

TIRED
AF

GIVE A
DAMN

FUCKING
TGIF

GIVE A
DAMN

FUCKING
TGIF

GIVE A
DAMN

FUCKING
TGIF

FUCKING
TGIF

FUCKING
TGIF

GIVE A
DAMN

FUCKING
PUT ON
PANTS
TODAY

SHIT
HAPPENS

FIERCE
AS FUCK

SHIT
HAPPENS

DIDN'T
FUCKING
CRY
TODAY

FUCKING
PUT ON
PANTS
TODAY

DIDN'T
FUCKING
CRY
TODAY

FIERCE
AS FUCK

SHIT
HAPPENS